How to Start a Vegan Diet

The Basics of Vegan Eating, Weight Loss, And Muscle Building

Wait! Before You Begin… Are You A Vegan Looking To Lose A Few Pounds And Get In Shape ?

If you answered YES then you are not alone. It is no secret that almost everyone wants to get in shape, build muscle, and look great. Unfortunately, most of us have no idea how to do it or where to even start! Yes- dieting and quick trips to the gym can work; but doing it wrong can lead to frustration and failure.

If you were hoping to find fitness tips tailor-made for your vegan lifestyle- then you've found the right place! Right now, you can get full **FREE access to 4 VEGAN FITNESS AND LIFESTYLE GUIDES.** These four reports are filled with crucial vegan fitness tips, hacks, and secrets! Become an instant vegan fitness pro after reading this book and these **FREE GUIDES!**

BuffVeggie.com

Download 4 Of the Best Beginner Vegan Fitness and Health Guides to Help You Get in Shape Fast 100% FREE!

Vegan Healthy Lifestyle -Learn More Vegan Tips and Tricks

Beginner's Guide to Plant-Based Fitness

100 Weight Loss Tips

Strategies That Guarantee Weight Loss for Life

CLICK HERE FOR INSTANT ACCESS
http://bit.ly/2uoLbuM

Table of Contents

INTRODUCTION

I want to not only thank you, but congratulate you for downloading this book, "How to Start a Vegan Diet, The Basics of Vegan Eating, Weight Loss, And Muscle Building."

Are you feeling overwhelmed, unhealthy, and unhappy? Do you feel as though getting fit and healthy is impossible? Have you found it hard to find comprehensive help online from other like-minded vegans? Would your life be better if you felt healthier and more in-shape? You may be under the impression that if you go vegan you will be nutrient deficient, weak, and unhealthy. However, you couldn't be more wrong! What you need are the basics to get you going. A vegan diet can be one of the most rewarding diets out there if you do it correctly.

This book will get you started towards accomplishing your goal of becoming a healthy vegan. Inside you will find proven information about the vegan diet (foods to eat and avoid, the benefits of being vegan, how to solve common risks), how this diet helps to lose weight, how a vegan diet helps build muscle, 10 protein-packed recipes, and finally some complementary bonus recipes!

I know what it's like to eat vegan and see no results in my weight or muscle. I would drag myself into the gym every single day and give it my all but I still saw no results. At one point I gave up, I figured being vegan meant I couldn't get the right amount of protein to build muscle or I would be too weak to lose weight. However, that all changed when I fixed my nutrition.

Most amazing bodies are built through proper nutrition, not by working out three hours a day. A vegan diet is special however. We need to be creative with how we get our protein and other nutrients- which is exactly what this book will show you.

Through following and applying the recipes and techniques found in this book- I guarantee you will start to see a positive change in your body. That is because these recipes are packed with protein and provide more than enough nutrients to keep you healthy. These fundamentals of a healthy vegan diet have not only worked for me, but for thousands of others who have tried them and have seen permanent success.

Thanks again for purchasing this book, I hope you enjoy it!

Clark Johnson

clarifying purposes only and are the owned by the owners themselves, not affiliated with this document.

WHAT IS A VEGAN DIET?

Simply speaking, a Vegan diet is a diet where an individual tries to exclude any and all form of produce and edible product that comes from animals such as meat. This also includes other products that come from animals such as milk or eggs.

To its followers, going vegan means more than just following a diet, it is a lifestyle. Many support the Vegan diet in hopes of abolishing animal cruelty and exploitation from the planet.

Now keep in mind, there is a difference between being a Vegetarian and being a vegan.

As mentioned earlier, veganism involves the complete expulsion of any kind of dairy/animal product from one's diet. However, vegetarianism allows some degree of freedom to the diet and often allows animal-derived products such as milk and egg.

Keep in mind that this book has been designed to illustrate the Vegan lifestyle specifically.

Different Types of Vegan

The different types of diets usually help people of different mindsets choose the one that best fits their preferred lifestyle.

Some of the more prominent ones include:

Whole food Vegan Diet: this is a diet that is based on a wide variety of different (whole) plant foods such as seeds, nuts, legumes, vegetables, fruits and whole grains.

Raw-Food Vegan Diet: This diet is composed of raw fruits, nuts, vegetables, plant foods or seeds that are cooked under temperatures of 118 degree Fahrenheit.

80/10/10: This unique diet encourages an individual to rely on fat rich plants such as avocados and nuts and focuses more on raw fruits and tender greens. This diet is also known as "Fruitarian diet"

The Starch Solution: This is similar to the aforementioned Fruitarian diet with the exception that it focuses on cooked starches such as rice, potatoes and corn instead of raw fruits.

Raw Till 4: This is a low-fat diet that is a variation of the fruitarian and Starch Solution diet. In this diet, Raw fruits are consumed up until 4 PM, after which, the individual has the option to cook a nice plant based meal to end the day with.

Junk-Food Vegan Diet: This diet relies largely on mock meats and vegan compliant cheese, desserts and fries. Not to mention, other heavily processed vegan produces as well!

Despite the differences in such types of Vegan diets- the core objective still remains the same.

"Get rid of meat, go for the greens!"

General Rules of Thumb

However, if you are not interested in following any of those types of diet, then as a rule of thumb, you should try to adhere by the following general guidelines in order to qualify as a vegan and start your journey.

Try to eat at least five portions of many different fruits and veggies a day

Make sure to keep your base meals circled around rice, bread, potatoes, pasta and other starchy carbs.

Go for dairy alternatives such as soya drinks, yogurt and other low fat/low sugar options.

Try to pack in some nuts and beans to ensure that you are supplied with protein.

If using oil and spreads, make sure to go for unsaturated ones, in small portions.

Make sure to keep yourself packed with lots of water preferably 6-8 cups per day.

Clark Johnson

Vegan Food Roadmap

Here is a brief outline of the different types of foods that you are allowed to gobble up!

Tofu, Seitan and Tempeh: These are excellent providers of proteins and are rich alternatives to fish, poultry and meat.

Legumes: These include beans, peas and lentils, which are also great sources of many essential nutrients and beneficial plant compounds.

Nuts and Nut Butters: Go for pure unroasted and unblanched ones as they are packed with selenium, zinc, fiber, iron etc.

Seeds: Flaxseed, hemp and chia are good choices when it comes to seeds as they are packed with a good dose of omega-3 fatty acids and protein.

Algae: Chlorella and Spirulina are good choices when it comes to seeking out good sources of protein-packed Algae.

Calcium-Fortified Plant Milks and Yogurts: These are excellent alternatives for a Vegan to meet their daily recommended calcium intake.

Nutritional Yeast: Make sure to go for the ones that are labeled "Vitamin B12" as they are fortified for maximum benefit.

Sprouted and Fermented Plant Foods: Produces such as tempeh, natto, miso, pickles, kombucha and Kimchi fall under this category, and they offer a good amount of vitamin K2 and probiotics.

Whole Grain Cereals and Pseudocereals: These are good providers of complex carbs, iron and Vitamin B.

Vegetables and Fruits: These should make up the bulk of your diet. They are amazing sources of nutrients and leafy greens including bok choy, kale, mustard greens and even spinaches are jam-packed with calcium and iron.

Food to avoid

Alternatively, these are the products, which you should refrain yourself from.

Meat: Lamb, beef, horse, veal, organ meat, chicken, wild meat, goose, turkey, quail, duck etc.

Fish and Seafood: All types of sea food are restricted including squid, shrimp, anchovies, calamari, crab etc.

Eggs: Any kind of eggs, including ostrich, quail, chicken, and fish are off the table.

Dairy: Ice Cream, cheese, cream, milk, butter etc are restricted.

Animal-Based Produce and Ingredients: For example: whey, lactose, casein, egg white albumen, carmine, gelatin etc. are to be avoided.

Bee Products: Such as royal jelly, pollen, honey etc. are to be avoided as well.

Now if this is your first time trying to go on a Vegan diet, the above-mentioned list might discourage you to some extent. But don't let it! The advantages of being a Vegan more than make up for the sacrifices that are made!

Amazing Advantages of Becoming a Vegan

Protection from various chronic diseases such as Type 2 Diabetes

Greatly reduces the possibility of suffering from cardiovascular diseases or Ischemic heart diseases

Relieves your stress and keeps you free from hypertension

Lowers the possibility of you suffering from a stroke

Helps to prevent obesity

Protects you against various cancers, including colon and prostate

Increases the health of your bones, preventing arthritis

Increases your kidney functionality

Helps prevent the development of Alzheimer's

And that is just the tip of the iceberg!

How to Solve Common Vegan Risks

As a Vegan, you must learn to appreciate the fact that an individual cannot expect to stay completely healthy just by eating a bucket of vegetables every day!

In fact, a properly prepared diet plan is essential to ensure that the body is well provided with nutrient-rich content, as otherwise it will start to suffer from deficiencies.

Since Vegans tend to replace all (if not most) processed foods with plant-based alternatives; they are a larger risk of suffering from Vitamin B12, Vitamin 2, Omega 3, Iron, Iodine, Zinc and Calcium deficiencies.

Therefore, a proper diet is a must. So make sure to keep the following points in mind:

Make sure to include foods that are fortified with calcium, vitamin B12 and Vitamin D on your plate. Examples include fortified almond, rice milk, soy, orange juice, collard greens, turnip, bok choy, dried figs etc.

Try to ferment sprouts and cook your food in order to enhance absorption of zinc and iron

Make sure to use iron cast pots and pans while cooking to avoid messy clean ups after cooking.

A little bit of iodized salt or seaweed will help maintain appropriate iodine levels

For Omega-3, go for chia, flaxseeds, soybeans, hemp etc.

Supplements

Vegans are allowed to take supplements to make up for their deficiencies. Sometimes it becomes tough for an individual to properly follow all of the rules.

The below supplements should be kept in mind in order to make sure that you are getting a proper vegan diet. You should choose them to be your daily nutrient drivers.

Vitamin B12: Try to take supplements that contain B12 in cyanocobalamin form for maximum effectiveness.

Vitamin D: Go for D2 or Vegan D3 that are manufactured by Viridian or Nordic Naturals.

Iron: Should only be ingested via means of supplements if you should have a deficiency. Otherwise, avoid taking extra Iron.

EPA and DHA: Take from algae oil.

Iodine: Either take supplements or add ½ a teaspoon of iodized salt to your daily diet.

Zinc: Take in forms of Zinc Citrate or Zinc Gluconate. Make sure that you don't take these while taking Calcium supplements.

Calcium: Take tablets of 500mg or less daily.

A note for pregnant or breastfeeding individuals

It should be noted that during breastfeeding or pregnancy, Vegan women are not strictly required to follow a Vegan diet- as a proper amount of nutrients are needed to supply the baby and encourage healthy development.

Clark Johnson

So, if you are indeed bringing up a baby, make sure that you consume a wide variety of different foods in order to make sure that your baby is getting enough vitamins and nutrients for adequate growth.

HOW BEING VEGAN HELPS YOU LOSE WEIGHT

A recent study found in the Journal of General Internal Medicine proved that going vegan worked very well for losing weight.

The researchers put their best food forward during the study and analyzed with great depth 12 different diets that included the Atkins, the American Diatheses Association Diet and so on.

Amongst the dozen, a Vegan diet proved to be the best.

The results astonished the scientists when they found out that it is possible to lose more than 5 pounds of weight when following a Vegan diet as opposed to only a few pounds lost on other more mainstream diets.

This was a significant leap from the other diets in the research.

The Science Behind the Diet

Curious to know why a Vegan Diet works so well?

The answer lies in the fiber!

There are actually two different types of fiber- and fiber doesn't really help to burn fat, rather it acts as a catalyst, which helps you to increase the rate at which you burn fat through other activities.

Soluble

Insoluble

When you are constantly on a diet that contains a plethora of insoluble fiber-rich foods, the fiber tends to work as a form of bulldozer to clear out the intestines of unnecessary leftovers... thus making you feel cleaner and healthier.

Alternatively, soluble fiber helps to eliminate fat and lower cholesterol by preventing the rapid absorption of sugar and fat into the blood stream.

This helps you get a steady stream of energy all throughout the day while burning up the fat, and prevents sugar spikes as well.

This, alongside the fact that eating a good amount of Fibrous fruits and vegetables will help you to feel full, will greatly help you to stay away from fatty foods (or foods in general) and you will eventually start to trim down fat on the go.

Tips on How to Lose Weight

By now you have already understood that veganism won't directly help you trim down your weight, rather it will indirectly help you to burn excess fats.

Aside from eating fiber-rich veggies and fruits, the following tips will greatly increase the effectiveness of your diet!

When undergoing a vegan transformation, initially it will be really hard to resist the temptation of meat. Therefore, it is of the utmost importance that you build up a very strong mental mindset that you are not allowed to eat meat. Embrace the absence of meat head-on. This will make your vegan journey easier.

Don't increase your intake of desserts and breads just because they are "Vegan compliant". Cut them down to one portion, and especially avoid sodas!

Try to go for high-protein and low-fat smoothies in order to keep your muscles pumped up- avoid fruit juices. They will help to gush the essential nutrients faster. Just make sure to replace the base milk with non-dairy products such as unsweetened soy milk.

Make sure to cut back on your sugar intake too; as it will make it much harder for you to lose weight.

If your plan is to lose weight, then go for green leafy vegetables such as Bok Choy, Collard Greens, etc. They will provide you with a good dose of calcium, which will make your weight loss effort more efficient.

Keep in mind that simply eating veggies won't trim down your weight if you just sit around all day! Try to get some aerobic exercise in order to maximize your effort. Even a 30-minute treadmill walk will do! Just make sure to do a warm up session of 15 minutes before starting your exercise.

What to Do If You Can't Lose Weight

In some unfortunate cases, an individual who has been going through a Vegan diet for a really long time might actually end up gaining more weight than losing it!

The main reason for this is a general lack of control over the vegan palette which the person is eating.

If you are aiming to go Vegan to lose weight, make sure to keep the following things in mind:

Control your portions. Just because the food is healthy, doesn't mean that you should go overboard! Maintain a balance and don't overeat anything.

Make sure to keep yourself supplied with protein. (We will be discussing this in depth in the next chapter).

Make sure to eat your meals on time. You cannot have your breakfast at noon and dinner in the morning!

Avoid plant-based junk foods such as coconut milk ice cream or sweetened potato chips! They won't do you any good.

Make sure to avoid high calorie beverages. Drinking chia drinks, almond milk, coffee brews, and green juices are good examples. If you don't want to avoid them, then control your input and don't drink more than one glass per day. However, the best method would be to drink lots of water, but if you need something sweet then opt for smoothies instead of juices.

Vegetables and Fruits for Weight Loss

These are some of the best fruits and veggies that you would want to consume to encourage your weight loss.

Broccoli

Green/Red Peppers

Spinach

Pickles

Potatoes

Onions

Black Beans

Avocado

Oats

Blueberries

Pears

Grapefruit

Kidney Beans

Almonds

Lentils

Banana

Orange

Pine Nuts

White Beans

3

THE SECRET BEHIND VEGAN MUSCLE BUILDING

While most are happy with and look to achieve a trimmed-out belly and a healthy lifestyle, there are others who prefer to take things up a notch and tone their body by building muscle.

Before moving forward, let me clarify that there is actually a huge misconception that muscles cannot be properly developed while on a Vegan diet!

Four-time Mr. Universe Bill Pearl, Ultimate Fighting Champion Mac Danzig and triathlete Brendan Brazier all are vegans! They can all be looked upon as symbols of true inspiration when it comes to building a toned body while being on a vegan diet.

Aside from your regular muscle-building routine, there are certain key aspects of a vegan diet which you should keep in mind in order to ensure that your muscles are developing properly.

However, it all comes down to just a single macronutrient…Protein!

Essential Nutrients You Need to Know

These are the nutrients which we consume to provide the energy required for our cells.

Protein: This is also known as the "building block of the body" since it helps to generate and heal different kinds of tissues in our body. It promotes growth and development.

Fat: While people often look at fat in a negative way, it is also essential as it acts as a backup reservoir of energy for the body.

Carbohydrates: Carbohydrates are the primary source of energy in our body. They range from simple to complex and are often very easily converted to energy.

Water: Water helps to maintain the optimum level of homeostasis in our body and is responsible for allowing the body to easily transport nutrients all around itself.

Minerals: Aside from the main nutrients, there are essential minerals that are needed in trace amounts in order to maintain a healthy body. For example, Potassium helps to maintain optimum cell fluid level, calcium strengthens the bones and so on.

Vitamins: Similar to minerals, vitamins are also needed in trace amounts to ensure that the body is functioning properly. Having a lack of certain vitamins often leads to severe health problem. For example, Vitamin C is responsible for collagen synthesis, which helps to maintain the blood structure; on the other hand, Vitamin D helps to ensure that the body's calcium homeostasis level is maintained correctly.

Clark Johnson

The Basics of Protein

As you can already tell, protein is at the core of building your muscle. You will soon find out that meat is not the only source of good protein that is out there!

You must learn to appreciate the quality and effectiveness of protein. It is determined by a value that is called "Protein Digestibility-Corrected Amino Acid Score" (PDCAAS), which essentially compares the quality of protein amino acid with the requirements of a human and the ability of a human to digest it.

Eggs for example have a very high PDCAAS count, but since vegans are not allowed to eat eggs, it is essential that you know about different sources through which you will be able to get your protein.

To give you a rough example, a 200lb bodybuilder would require about 200g of protein every day. This is because bodybuilders usually require one gram of protein per pound of weight every day to encourage proper growth.

Animal Vs. Plant Protein

There has been a long-standing debate between these two types of protein and their effectiveness when it comes to muscle building.

Perhaps the core difference between animal and plant protein comes from the essential amino acids that are required by the body.

Animal proteins such as meat, eggs or dairy are similar in nature to human beings' natural protein; thus, they are very easily absorbed. However, they are also high in LDL cholesterol and saturated fat, which might lead to harmful consequences in the long run.

Plant protein on the other hand is actually rather similar to animal protein, with the absence of just one or two essential amino acids for the body.

In terms of nutritional values, animal proteins tend to be very high in saturated fat and low in dietary fiber. Red meats have also been linked to a number of different health issues such as heart diseases and cancer.

Alternatively, plant-based proteins tend to be lower in sodium and higher in fiber!

However, the problem when answering the question, "is vegan protein suitable for body building?" generally arises due to the difference between the amount of protein available in animal and plant protein.

For example, a cut of steak will provide you with approximately 40g of protein. Alternatively, a cup of tempeh will provide you with 31g of protein.

The answer to the question ultimately boils down to, "are you able to fulfill your daily protein intake (for body building) relying solely on vegetables?"

Clark Johnson

The answer is yes.

You might need to consume veggies in a more balanced and proper way; but it is indeed possible.

Fruits and Veggies That Have Lots of Protein

Organic Edamame: 18 per cup

Organic Tempeh: 16g per 3 ounces

Organic Tofu: 8-15g per 3 ounces

Lentils: 9g per 1/2 cup

Black Beans: 7.6g per 1/2 cup

Lima Beans: 7.3g per 1/2 cup

Peanuts/ Peanut Butter: 7g per 1/4 cup

Wild Rice: 6.5g per 1 cup

Chickpeas: 6g

Almonds: 6g

Chia Seeds:6g per 2 tablespoons

Steep Cut Oatmeal:5g of 1/4 cup

Cashews: 5g per 1/4 cup

Pumpkin Seeds: 5g per 1/4 cup

Potatoes: 4g in 1 white potato (medium)

Spinach: 3g per 1/2 a cup

Organic Corn:2.5g per 1/2 cup

Avcado:2g per 1/2 of an avocado

Broccoli: 2g per 1/2 a cup

Brussels Sprouts: 2g per 1/2 cup

Where to Find the Other Nutrients You Need

Aside from consuming protein and working out, you should also maintain your fat and carbohydrate levels to properly ensure that your muscles are building up properly.

Fats: Fat is an extremely essential macronutrient that is required to provide energy to the body. But in terms of body building, a bodybuilder needs about 0.5g of fat per pound. So, following our previous example, a 200-pound bodybuilder would require about 100g of fat to properly develop muscles. However, 70g-80g should suffice as well.

Good sources of vegan fat include:

Seeds such as hemp, sunflower seeds, chia seeds etc.

Coconut oil

Avocados

Cacao Nibs

Nuts

Carbohydrates: Carbohydrates are required to provide the body with energy to fuel those intense training sessions. Lowering down on your carbohydrate intake would result in fatigue and lethargy; resulting in you not being able to exercise properly at all!

Good sources of vegan carbohydrates include:

Whole fruits

Lentils

Unprocessed Starchy Veggies such as Winter Squash, Whole corn and Sweet Potatoes

Beans

Quinoa

Lentils

Whole Grains such as Oats, Barley, Brown Rice etc.

To sum things up, as a general rule of thumb, aside from your strength exercise, you should keep in mind the following points:

Make sure to break down your total protein intake into 5-6 small sized meals per day. Each meal should have a large variety of fruits, whole grains, nuts, water and vegetables.

Make sure that more than half of your daily calories come from quality carbohydrates.

Make sure to not cut down on fats as they are required to supply energy to the body while intense workout sessions occur.

And last but the not the least; if possible, do consult with a registered nutritionist who might be able to help you create a personalized vegan diet plan that will complement your workout session.

If you are extracting value from this book so far, it would help me tremendously if you would be kind enough to leave me a review.

Click Here to Leave a Review on Amazon!

https://www.amazon.com/review/create-review/ref=dpx_acr_wr_link?asin=B074RSYND1

4

10 VEGAN PROTEIN RECIPES

Creamy Vegan Fettuccine Alfredo with Lemon Dashes

Ingredients:

12 ounces of eggless fettuccine

2 cups of unsweetened soy milk

4 ounces of soy cream cheese

3 tablespoons of blanched and sliced almonds

3 tablespoons of nutritional yeast

1 teaspoon of finely grated lemon zest

Kosher salt as needed

Ground black pepper as needed

2 tablespoons of extra virgin olive oil

3 finely chopped garlic cloves

1/2 cup of loosely packed parsley leaves, chopped up

Preparation:

Step 1: Take a large sized pot and fill it up with water

Step 2: Bring the water to a boil and add in fettuccine

Step 3: Cook the fettuccine until it is firm

Step 4: Make sure to keep 1 cup of cooking water for use later

Step 5: Open up the lid of your blender and add soy milk, almonds, soy cream cheese, nutritional yeast, 1 teaspoon of salt, lemon zest and 1/4 teaspoon of pepper

Step 6: Blend the whole mixture well

Step 7: Take a large-sized skillet and place it on the stove at medium heat

Step 8: Add oil and heat it up

Step 9: Add garlic and stir-cook it for 1 minute

Step 10: Add the blended soy milk mixture into the skillet and 1/2 cup of your reserved cooking liquid from the pasta- cook for about 8 minutes until the mixture is creamy and thick

Step 11: Remove the heat

Step 12: Add your cooked fettuccini to the mix alongside parsley

Step 13: Give the whole mixture a toss

Step 14: Sprinkle a bit of yeast and grind some pepper on top

Step 15: Serve!

Nutrition Values
Protein: 22g
Carbs: 74g
Fats: 15g
Calories: 520
Dietary Fiber: 6g

Fresh and Fit Red Onion and Kale Pasta

Ingredients:

2 and 1/2 cups of vegetable broth

3/4 cup of dry lentils

1/2 a teaspoon of salt

1 bay leaf

1/4 cup of olive oil

1 large sized chopped up red onion

1 teaspoon of chopped fresh thyme

1/2 a teaspoon of chopped up fresh oregano

1/2 a teaspoon of salt

1/2 a teaspoon of black pepper

8 ounces of vegan sausage sliced up into 1/4-inch slices

1 bunch of coarsely chopped kale with stems removed

1 pack of rotini

2 tablespoons of nutritional yeast

Preparation:

Step 1: Take a saucepan and place it over a high heat

Step 2: Add vegetable broth, 1/2 a teaspoon of salt, lentils, and the bay leaf- then bring the mixture to a boil

Step 3: Lower the heat to medium-low and cover it up

Step 4: Let it cook for about 20 minutes until the lentils are tender

Step 5: Add some more broth if required, remove the bay leaf

Step 6: Take another skillet and place it over medium-high heat, add olive oil and heat it up

Step 7: Stir in onion, oregano, thyme, 1/2 a teaspoon of salt, and pepper

Step 8: Cook for about 1 minute

Step 9: Add the Vegan sausage and lower the heat down to medium-low

Step 10: Cook for about 10 minutes until the onions are tender

Step 11: Take a large pot and fill it up with salted water

Step 12: Bring the water to a boil over a high heat

Step 13: Add rotini pasta and kale

Step 14: Cook for about 8 minutes until firm

Step 15: Remove a bit of the cooking water and keep it on the side for later use

Step 16: Drain the pasta and return it to the pot

Step 17: Stir in your lentils mixture alongside the onion mix

Step 18: Add the reserved cooking water to add just a bit of moistness

Step 19: Sprinkle a bit of yeast and serve!

Nutrition Values
Protein: 36g
Carbs: 111g
Fats: 16g
Calories: 732
Dietary Fiber: 19g

Italian Tofu Parmigiana

Ingredients:

1/2 cup of seasoned bread crumbs

5 tablespoons of grated Vegan Parmesan cheese (recipe provided below)

2 teaspoons of dried oregano

Salt as needed

Ground black pepper as needed

1 pack of firm tofu

2 tablespoons of olive oil

1 can of tomato sauce

1/2 a teaspoon of dried basil

1 minced garlic clove

4 ounces of mozzarella cheese (recipe provided below)

Preparation:

Step 1: Take a small sized bowl and add in bread crumbs, 2 tablespoons of Parmesan cheese, salt, black pepper, 1 teaspoon of oregano

Step 2: Slice up your tofu into 1/4-inch-thick slices and add it into a bowl of cold water

Step 3: Press the tofu slices gently into your bread crumb mixture and turn them well to coat them on all sides (one at a time)

Step 4: Take a medium-sized skillet and place it over a medium heat, add oil and then heat it up

Step 5: Add the covered tofu and cook it until it's crispy on just one side. Add olive oil and turn it over, make the other side crispy and brown as well

Step 6: Take an 8-inch square baking pan

Step 7: Grab a bowl and add tomato sauce, oregano, basil and garlic

Step 8: Mix well and pour it in your baking pan as a single layer

Step 9: Arrange your cooked tofu slices in the pan, drizzle sauce on the tofu

Step 10: Top it off with your mozzarella and 3 tablespoons of Parmesan

Step 11: Bake for about 20 minutes at 400 degrees Fahrenheit

Step 12: Serve!

Nutrition Values
Protein: 25g
Carbs: 18g
Fats: 21g
Calories: 357
Dietary Fiber: 3.9g

Clark Johnson

Vegan Bangin' Burritos

Ingredients:

3/4 cup of white rice

1 and a 1/2 cup of water

1 pack of frozen soy burger style crumbles

1 can of whole tomatoes (drained with 1/4 cup of juice reserved)

2 and a 1/2 teaspoons of chili powder

1 teaspoon of cumin

1 pack of taco seasoning mix

2 (10 inch sized) burrito sized flour tortillas

1 can of vegetarian refried beans

2 pieces of seeded, divided and sliced jalapeno peppers

1 and a 1/2 cup of salsa

2 and a 1/2 cups of shredded cheddar cheese

Preparation:

Step 1: Take a saucepan and add water

Step 2: Bring the water to a boil

Step 3: Add rice and keep stirring it

Step 4: Lower down the heat and let it simmer for about 20 minutes

Step 5: Pre-heat your oven to a temperature of 375-degrees Fahrenheit

Step 6: Take a medium-sized frying pan and add soy crumbles, reserved tomato juice, tomatoes, chili powder, taco seasoning and cumin- then place it over a medium-high heat

Step 7: Cook for about 10 minutes, making sure to break up the tomatoes

Step 8: Take an 8x8inch baking dish (greased) and lay 1 flour tortilla in it

Step 9: Layer it up with one half of your beans, rice, jalapeño slices, soy mixture and just 1 cup of cheddar cheese

Step 10: Keep repeating the process until all of the ingredients are used

Step 11: Top it up with another 1 and a ½ cups of cheddar cheese

Step 12: Bake in your oven for about 15 minutes until the cheese has melted well

Step 13: Serve!

Nutrition Values
Protein: 50g
Carbs: 486g
Fats: 18g
Calories: 486
Dietary Fiber: 7.7g

Clark Johnson

Festive Black Bean Croquettes and Fresh Salsa

Ingredients:

2 cans of 15-ounce black beans (rinsed)	1/4 cup of chopped fresh cilantro
1 teaspoon of ground cumin	1 teaspoon of chili powder (if you want it to be spicy)
1/4 cup of plain dry breadcrumbs	1/4 teaspoon of salt
2 cups of finely chopped tomatoes	1 tablespoon of extra virgin olive oil
2 sliced scallions	1 diced avocado

Preparation:

Step 1: Pre-heat your oven to a temperature of 425 degrees Fahrenheit

Step 2: Take a baking sheet and grease it up with cooking spray

Step 3: Take a large-sized bowl and mash black beans and cumin using a fork, do this until there are no whole-sized beans

Step 4: Take another medium-sized bowl and add tomatoes, cilantro, scallions, 1/2 a teaspoon of chili powder and salt- mix them well

Step 5: Stir in 1 cup of the tomato mix into the bowl with the black bean mix

Step 6: Take a small bowl and add 1/3 cup of breadcrumbs, 1/2 a teaspoon of chili powder and oil. Mix well until the breadcrumbs are fully coated

Step 7: Prepare the bean mixture into 8 1/2 cup balls

Step 8: Carefully press the balls into the breadcrumbs, making sure to turn them in order to coat them well. Transfer them onto your pre-prepared baking sheet

Step 9: Bake the croquettes for about 20 minutes in your oven until the breadcrumbs show a nice golden texture.

Step 10: Stir the avocado into your tomato mixture. Serve the salsa alongside the baked croquette

Step 11: Enjoy!

Nutrition Values
Protein: 16g
Carbs: 61g
Fats: 13g
Calories: 404
Dietary Fiber: 17g

Hearty Vegan Shepherd's Pie

Ingredients:

For the Mashed Potato Layer

5 pieces of russet potatoes peeled and cut up into 1-inch cubes

1/2 cup of vegan mayonnaise (recipe provided below)

1/2 cup of soy milk

1/4 cup of olive oil

3 tablespoons of vegan cream cheese substitute (similar to Tofutti)

2 teaspoons of salt

For the Bottom Layer

1 tablespoon of vegetable oil

1 large sized onion chopped up

2 chopped up carrots

3 chopped up celery stalks

1 chopped up tomato

1 minced garlic clove

1 teaspoon of Italian seasoning

A pinch of ground black pepper

1 pack of vegetarian ground beef substitute

1/2 cup of shredded cheddar style soy cheese

Preparation:

Step 1: Take a pot and add in the potatoes

Step 2: Fill it up with cold water

Step 3: Bring the water to a boil over medium-high heat

Step 4: Bring it down to a low heat and keep boiling the potatoes for about 25 minutes until they are soft

Step 5: Stir in the soy milk, vegan mayonnaise, olive oil, vegan cream cheese, and salt into the potato mix

Step 6: Mash up the potatoes using a potato masher until the whole mixture is smooth and fluffy

Step 7: Transfer it onto a plate and let it sit

Step 8: Pre-heat your oven to 400 degrees Fahrenheit

Step 9: Take a 2-quart baking dish and grease it up with cooking spray

Step 10: Take a large-sized skillet and place it over a medium heat

Step 11: Add vegetable oil and heat it up

Step 12: Add onions, celery, carrots, frozen peas, and tomato

Step 13: Cook them for about 10 minutes until they are tender

Step 14: Stir in garlic, pepper and Italian seasoning

Step 15: Lower the heat to medium-low and crumble in the vegan ground beef substitute

Step 16: Cook for about 5 minutes to ensure that it is broken up well

Step 17: Spread the vegan meat mix onto the bottom part of your baking dish

Step 18: Top it with mashed potato mix

Step 19: Smoothen it so that it evens out the layer

Step 20: Sprinkle in your potatoes with shredded soy cheese

Step 21: Bake in your pre-heated oven for about 20 minutes until the casserole is hot and shows a slightly brown texture

Step 22: Serve!

Nutrition Values
Protein: 20g
Carbs: 64g
Fats: 24g
Calories: 552
Dietary Fiber: 6.6g

Garden Gourmet Squash, Gnocchi, Spinach, And Chickpea Platter

Ingredients:

1 pound of frozen gnocchi	2 tablespoons of currants
1 tablespoon of extra virgin olive oil	1 tablespoon of freshly chopped sage
2 cups of thinly-sliced and peeled butternut squash	1/4 a teaspoon of freshly ground black pepper
1/2 a cup of sliced shallots	8 cups of fresh spinach (coarsely chopped)
2 cloves of minced garlic	
1 can of 14-ounce vegetable broth	1 can of 15-ounce chickpeas
	1/4 cup of balsamic vinegar

Preparation:

Step 1: Take a large pot and fill it up with water

Step 2: Bring the water to a boil and cook the gnocchi according to the instructions on the packet

Step 3: Drain the gnocchi and rinse it. Pat it dry using a clean towel.

Step 4: Take a large non-stick skillet and place it over a medium heat

Step 5: Add gnocchi and cook it slowly until it starts to brown for about 5-7 minutes. Take another bowl and transfer the cooked gnocchi to that bowl

Clark Johnson

Step 6: Add 1 teaspoon of oil, shallots, squash and garlic to the pan and stir fry them for about 2 minutes. Stir in sage, pepper, broth and currants- then bring the mixture to a boil

Step 7: Lower down the heat and let the mixture simmer and keep cooking it for about 6-8 minutes until the squash is thoroughly cooked

Step 8: Add chickpeas, spinach and gnocchi to the broth as well and cook them for an additional 2 minutes to ensure that the spinach has wilted

Step 9: Serve with a drizzle of balsamic vinegar

Note: If you are using shelf-stable gnocchi, then you can skip steps 1-5 and go directly to step 6

Nutrition Values
Protein: 15g
Carbs: 92g
Fats: 6g
Calories: 485
Dietary Fiber: 9g

Tasty Tofu Squash Curry

Ingredients:

2 tablespoons of curry powder

1/2 a teaspoon of salt

1/4 teaspoon of freshly ground pepper

1 pack of 14 ounce extra firm tofu

3 teaspoons of canola oil

1 large-sized delicate squash halved and seeded. Cut up into 1-inch cubes

1 medium-sized sliced and halved onion

2 teaspoons of grated fresh ginger

1 can of 14-ounce coconut milk

1 teaspoon of light brown sugar

8 cups of chopped kale, stem removed

1 tablespoon of lime juice

Preparation:

Step 1: Take a small bowl and add curry powder, pepper and salt

Step 2: Blot the tofu dry using a clean kitchen towel and cut it up into 1-inch cubes

Step 3: Take a medium sized bowl and toss the tofu pieces with 1 teaspoon of your prepared spice mixture

Step 4: Take a large skillet and place it over a medium-high heat. Heat up 2 teaspoons of oil

Step 5: Add tofu and cook for about 6-8 minutes, making sure to give it a stir after every 2 minutes.

Step 6: Transfer the tofu onto a plate

Step 7: Add 2 teaspoons of oil over medium-high heat again and add squash, ginger, onion and the rest of your spice mixture

Step 8: Stir fry them for about 4-5 minutes until the veggies are fully browned

Step 9: Add coconut milk and brown sugar and bring the mixture to a boil

Step 10: Add half of your kale and cook for about 1 minute

Step 11: Stir in the remaining greens and cook for another 1 minute

Step 12: Return the tofu to this pan and cook for about 3-5 minutes, making sure to mix the whole mixture once or twice in order to ensure that the squash and greens are tender

Step 13: Remove the heat and squeeze a bit of lime juice on

Step 14: Serve!

Nutrition Values
Protein: 16g
Carbs: 29g
Fats: 18g
Calories: 316
Dietary Fiber: 8g

Authentic Indian Lentils, Rosemary And Greens On Warm Bread

Ingredients:

3 cloves of garlic

2 tablespoons of extra virgin olive oil

1/2 a teaspoon of crushed red pepper

2 tablespoons of tomato paste

2 teaspoons of chopped fresh rosemary

4 cups of water

1 cup of French green lentils

8 cups of chopped kale

3/4 teaspoon of kosher salt

4 slices of stale crusty bread

Preparation:

Step 1: Take a Dutch oven and place it over a medium heat

Step 2: Mince up 2 garlic cloves

Step 3: Add 2 tablespoons of oil to the Dutch oven and add the minced garlic alongside red pepper and cook them for about 1 minute

Step 4: Add water and bring the mixture to a boil

Step 5: Add lentils and lower down the heat to a simmer

Step 6: Partially cover the oven and cook for about 40 minutes

Step 7: Add kale and salt. Then cover it up and cook for about 10 minutes more until the kale and lentils are soft

Step 8: In the meantime, pre-heat your oven to a temperature of 375-degrees Fahrenheit

Step 9: Cut up the rest of your garlic clove in half and rub your toast with the garlic

Step 10: Serve each of your pieces of toast topped up with 1 cup of lentil mixture alongside a drizzle of 1/2 a teaspoon of oil

Note: To prepare the bread, bake the slices of bread at 250 degrees Fahrenheit until they are crispy for about 15-20 minutes.

Nutrition Values

Protein: 19g

Carbs: 57g

Fats: 15g

Calories: 425

Dietary Fiber: 12g

Savory Stir-Fried Noodles with Green Tea

Ingredients:

8 ounces of whole wheat noodles

2 tablespoons of canola oil

1 teaspoon of loose green tea leaves

2 teaspoons of minced fresh ginger

2 minced garlic cloves

8 ounces of flavored baked tofu, cut up into matchsticks

1 small sized red bell pepper cut up into thin strips

1 small sized yellow bell pepper cut up into thin strips

4 scallions cut up into 2-inch pieces

2 tablespoons of reduced sodium soy sauce

2 tablespoons of rice vinegar

1 teaspoon of toasted sesame oil

1/4 teaspoon of freshly ground pepper

Preparation:

Step 1: Take a pot and add water

Step 2: Bring the water to a boil and cook your noodles according to the package instructions

Step 3: Drain the noodles and rinse them with cold water

Step 4: Take a wok and place it over medium heat

Step 5: Add oil and swirl the wok to coat it well

Step 6: Add tea leaves, garlic and ginger- cook them for just 30 seconds until nicely fragrant

Clark Johnson

Step 7: Add tofu and cook for about 2 minutes

Step 8: Add yellow and red bell peppers and cook them for about 2 minutes until they are soft

Step 9: Stir in the noodles, soy sauce, scallions and vinegar

Step 10: Cook for about 2 minutes, making sure to keep stirring it from time to time

Step 11: Stir in pepper and sesame oil and toss well to combine it

Step 12: Serve warm!

Nutrition Values
Protein: 22g
Carbs: 47g
Fats: 16g
Calories: 421
Dietary Fiber: 5g

COMPLEMENTARY RECIPES

Simple Vegan Parmesan Cheese

Ingredients:

1/2 cup of blanched silvered almonds

1/2 cup of raw cashews

1/4 cup of nutritional yeast

1/2 teaspoon of kosher salt

1/4 teaspoon of garlic powder

Preparation:

Step 1: Take a food processor and add all of the listed ingredients

Step 2: Mix them well until a fine meal forms

Step 3: Store it and chill it in your fridge

Step 4: Sprinkle it on your dishes as you like

Step 5: As a side note, it can also be stored in your fridge for up to 2 months

Classic Vegan Mayonnaise

Ingredients:

1 clove of roasted garlic

A Pinch of salt

A Pinch of black pepper

3/4 tablespoon of Dijon mustard

1 and a 1/2 tablespoons of lemon juice

150ml of unsweetened Soya Milk

150ml of Sunflower oil

Preparation:

Step 1: Take a blender and add garlic, black pepper, salt, Dijon mustard, lemon juice and soy milk

Step 2: Mix them well and carefully pour the sunflower oil into the mix

Step 3: Add the mix into a jar and your mayo is ready!

Traditional Vegan Mozzarella Cheese

Ingredients:

2 cups of raw cashews (soaked overnight)

1 and 2/3 cup of hot water

6 tablespoons of tapioca starch

4 tablespoons of nutritional yeast

1 teaspoon of sea salt

1 tablespoon of lemon juice

Preparation:

Step 1: Take a blender and add all of the listed ingredients- blending them until you have the desired consistency (should be similar to milk)

Step 2: Take a large sized saucepan and place it over a medium heat

Step 3: Pour the contents of the blender into the pan and keep stirring well

Step 4: After a few minutes, it should start to thicken. Keep doing this for 10-15 minutes

Step 5: Remove the heat and wait for a few minutes

Step 6: Take a large bowl of water (cold) and add 1 tablespoon of salt

Step 7: Take an ice cream scoop and scoop up the mozzarella into balls

Step 8: Place the balls under cold water and keep them there for 1 minute

Clark Johnson

Step 9: Store the balls in the fridge for later use

CONCLUSION

I really want to thank you for reading this book. I sincerely hope you received value from it!

Like I said, this is the best information that led me to change my life and body. I followed what I put in this book, and I was able to lose weight and gain muscle. If you apply this knowledge towards your own life then I have no doubt you can start to see a positive change in your soul, mind, and body!

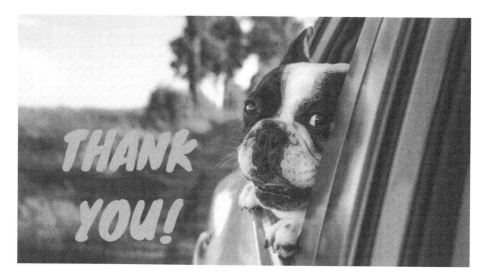

If you received value from this book, then I'd like to ask you for a favor. Would you be kind enough to leave a review for this book on Amazon?

Click Here to Leave a Review on Amazon!
https://www.amazon.com/review/create-review/ref=dpx_acr_wr_link?asin=B074RSYND1

I want to help as many people as I can with this book; more reviews will help me to accomplish that!

Thank you for your time, I wish you the best of luck on your vegan journey!

-Clark

Free Beginner's Guide to Plant-Based Fitness!

Take your knowledge to the next level. Expand on what you learned and start to take action. In this free guide, you will learn more recipes for a breakfast, lunch, dinner, and for snacking, what a vegan day may look like, and how to fix common mistakes at the gym. You will also be getting a free workout routine template to help you get started!

Click Here to Get Your Free Guide!

Preview:

One of the biggest sources of frustration many vegans and vegetarians have when it comes to their fitness and health is what in the world to do at the gym. Many instructors out there don't understand the intricacies of a plant-based diet; so their routines and programs are centered around heavy gains with lots of meat eating- yuck! Luckily for you, Buff Veggie is here to help you along your way!

A change you can make right away to how you approach working out is how much time you spend at the gym. Most of us correlate time spent at the gym with how much muscle we will gain- however this is simply not the case. The recommended time one should spend working out with weights (not cardio) is no more than 45 minutes. After that, your body is too exhausted and "beat up" to repair fully. Spending more time at the gym does not equal more results- focus on the fundamentals of your workouts and the results will come.

Continue reading in the free guide!

Get It *Here* http://bit.ly/2hSgcFU

For More Vegan Fitness Tips, Recipes, Cookbooks, Product Reviews, And Programs, Check Out buffveggie.com!

Learn about mistakes you need to correct in the gym, the best vitamin B12 supplement you should be taking, how becoming vegan can help your heart, and much, much more! Enjoy multiple articles each week that are aimed at getting you in the best possible shape while remaining 100% plant-based!

Check Out the Blog Here http://buffveggie.com/

Once again, thank you so much for reading this book! Good luck in all your future endeavors!

24903890R00035

Printed in Great Britain
by Amazon